MORE BEGINNER WORKOUTS: THE NEXT STEP

Training at Home with Basic Equipment

Book 2 in the Jade Mountain Workout Series

By Whit McClendon

Copyrights

More Beginner Workouts: The Next Step
Training at Home with Basic Equipment

Disclaimer:

ISBN-13: 978-0692078082 (Rolling Scroll Publishing)
ISBN-10: 0692078088

Cover Art by: Whit McClendon
Published by: Jade Mountain Martial Arts, Inc./Rolling Scroll Publishing, Katy, TX
Website: www.jmma.org

Acknowledgements

I've been learning and teaching martial arts and fitness concepts for over 30 years. Not only has it been exceedingly fun for me, but I've taken great pleasure in teaching others to enjoy the benefits of martial arts and fitness training. It has been deeply gratifying to hear back from students, even years later, thanking me for helping them get started on the path to a healthier lifestyle. As much as I've taught my many students, they have also taught me quite a bit. I've had some fabulous teachers both in martial arts and in the fitness industry, so I'd like to thank everyone who has ever spent time on the mats with me in any capacity. Without knowing it, you changed my life.

I've had a ton of support from my family, friends, colleagues, and students, and I appreciate them all. Thank you all so very much.

~Whit McClendon - 2018

Dedication

This book is dedicated to the people out there who are sick and tired of being sick and tired, and are willing to do something about it! I've met and worked with tons of folks who want to get in better physical shape but are nervous about getting started because they either don't know what to do or they think that they'll have to kill themselves to get fit. My heart has always gone out to people like that, and I want to help. If this book series can help even a single person to start exercising and live a healthier life, I will have succeeded.

Contents

Introduction

Hey, welcome back! If you've picked up this book, then you've probably read the first book in the Jade Mountain Workout Series, *Short Workouts for Beginners*, and you're ready for more!

By now, you're probably feeling accomplished; you've done the workouts from the first book, got started with those exercises and are now familiar with them, and maybe you're already feeling stronger and healthier! Congratulations! You've made a great start and taken some big steps on the road to being healthy, fit, and strong!

Now that you've got your feet under you, let's take it a step or two farther. Let's face it, changing up your workouts and exercises can make a big difference. Not only does changing up the exercises make your workouts more interesting, new movements also challenge your body to adapt in different ways that can improve your strength, balance, and coordination even more! That's definitely a good thing!

The exercises depicted in this book require a bit more from you than those in the previous book. You'll definitely be challenged by some or all of them! The good news is that you've got this. You can do it. Just give them a try and don't be afraid to mess up at first. Learn as you go, and just give it your best shot. Before you know it, you'll be ready for even bigger and better challenges!

As I always say, if you can't currently do all of the exercises perfectly, that's ok. Just strive to improve your technique each time and avoid hurting yourself. Do what you can with an eye toward working up to the other stuff that might be currently difficult. It's a learning process as well as a physical one, so don't beat yourself up as you start to "up your game;" just take it one step at a time.

Make sure you've talked to a doctor about your workout program, by the way. They'll probably be thrilled, but it's always good to get a checkup now and then, especially if it's been a while!

All right then, let's get you ready to work out!

Chapter 1 – Keeping Things Moving

Since this book is the second in the series, I'll assume that you've read the first one, and have tackled some or all of those workouts for some time now. You've become accustomed to the exercises, gotten used to working out, and are feeling stronger. You recover from your workouts faster, and you're starting to think you're ready for more challenging workouts.

That's awesome!

We covered the following points in the previous book, so I'll only touch on them with some additional comments this time.

1. **Get a checkup.** You should have checked with your doctor before you started exercising...you did that, right? You did? Great. Moving on.
2. **Get some sleep.** If you've been working out, then chances are that you've discovered one of the benefits of consistent exercise: better sleep. It's great! Folks often report that they're sleeping deeper, waking up less, and feeling generally better once they have created a habit of exercising. Here's the thing: even if you are sleeping fewer minutes, you REALLY need the sleep you get. Be sure to allow adequate time for sleep

so your body can recover from all your hard work and come back stronger.

3. **Drink more water!** Often, folks think they're hungry when their bodies are actually screaming for water. Get in the habit of staying hydrated. Remember that you're now an athlete, and you need to keep your body healthy and strong! Drink 2-3 liters of water a day.

4. **Eat the right stuff and avoid the junk.** There are lots of books out there on proper nutrition and hundreds of different approaches to healthy eating. As I said before, keep it simple. Eating lean meats and fish, fruits, and vegetables is a good plan. Go easy on the pasta and rice, but fist-sized portions of those foods are ok too. Watch your portion sizes and listen to your body. There's 'full,' and there's 'stuffed.' Stop eating when you're comfortably full and don't think you have to feel like a bloated water buffalo at the end of every meal. Remember: "You can't outwork a bad eating plan."

5. **Set yourself up to succeed.** By now, you've built some good habits. You've got your playlists set up, good shoes and workout clothes ready, and hopefully, you're used to blocking out some time to train. At this point, just

keep scheduling your workouts and sticking to your plan. You've got this.

6. **Don't obsess over the scale.** As I said before, it's just a number. The number doesn't describe how fit and amazing you are, only how much you weigh, so don't give it too much power.

7. **Take rest days.** Even when you consider yourself a solid athlete, you'll still need to take rest days. They are just as important to your overall health and fitness as workout days. Listen to your body, and rest when you feel like you need to (and then be sure to train the next day!). And don't train when you're sick. Running a fever? Diarrhea? Geez, get that handled first. Your body needs to use its resources to kick that sickness out before it can get back to business as usual, so take time off if you catch a bug.

The next chapter we'll talk about some basic, low-cost equipment you can purchase to increase the intensity of your workouts and bring about even better results.

Chapter 2 – Basic Equipment

While there are still tons of exercises that only require the use of your body and maybe a mat on the floor (and probably a towel to mop up the sweat), but if you've come this far, then you might be interested in picking up a few inexpensive pieces of equipment to improve your workouts. Also, I find that working with different pieces of equipment can make things interesting and fun because it adds variety to my workouts.

Because I really want readers to feel like this is something they can do even on a tight budget, I'm going to keep it simple, economical, and as easy as possible. Let's take a look at a few items that will help you whip yourself into even better shape.

1. Jump Rope – $5-$20 and up

There are lots of ropes available, many are adjustable, some are thick and heavy, some are thin and whippy, and you can still buy some that are actually made of rope or leather. I learned how to jump with an old Everlast leather jump rope that I absolutely wore out. I have a $40 custom steel-cable jumprope from Rogue that I like, but most of the time, I use a $4 plastic rope that feels great to me. Try out a few and pick something you think you'll like, then you'll know if you want to keep it or try something else.

The most important thing about a jump rope is the length. A good way to find out how long yours should be is to stand on the middle of the rope with one foot and pull the handles up in front of your chest (see picture). The ends of the rope should reach roughly to the middle of your sternum. Beginners usually do better with a slightly longer rope, and so you might want a few inches longer than that if your rope is adjustable. Most fixed ropes come in lengths of 7', 8', 9', etc.

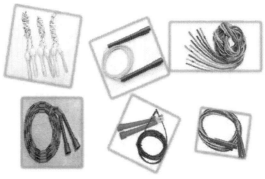

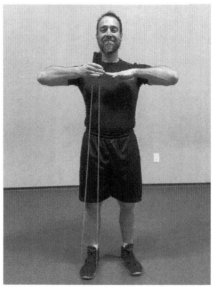

Measuring
your rope.

2. Medicine Ball – $15-$40 and up

Medicine Balls can be made of leather, rubber, or other synthetic. Medicine balls have been around in one form or other since ancient times, and commonly associated with boxers and fighters since the 1800's. You may not be training to be a fighter, but like them, you can certainly benefit from the increased core strength and joint stability that can come from medicine ball workouts! I suggest starting with a lighter ball, 6-10 lbs, before you try something heavier.

The workouts I will outline in this book can all be done indoors with a minimum of space, so you do not have to buy anything terribly expensive or specialized. Your local sporting goods store or department store likely has some decent options to get you started, and you can always order online.

I prefer rubber medicine balls (they resemble basketballs, just heavier!) because I can grip them easily and water (or sweat) won't damage them.

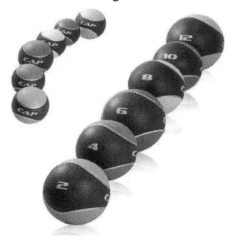
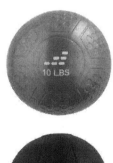
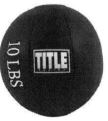

3. Pull-Up Bar – $17-$25 and up

When I mention pull-ups, lots of my students give me a "Have you gone crazy?" kind of look, since they may have not been able to do a pull-up since they were a kid. Never fear: we'll talk about how to get started with your pull-ups, no matter if you can currently do them or not. It's a process, right?

Unless you've outfitted your garage or other room in your house into a full-fledged gym, you likely do not have a permanent pull-up bar available. The doorway pull-up bar is a useful and convenient alternative. It fits right inside almost any doorway in your home and can be easily removed and put away when your workout is done. There are some obvious limitations with a device like this, but for most, it should suffice.

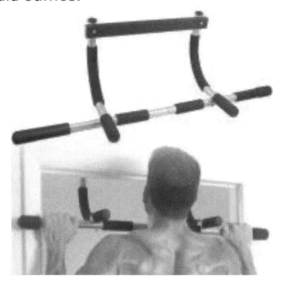

4. Other Stuff – There are tons of other pieces of equipment that could be used in your training: barbells, kettlebells, dumb bells, plyo boxes, stretch bands, and lots more. You will see many of these items detailed in later books, but for now, a jump rope, a medicine ball, and a doorway pull-up bar are the only things we will add to your workouts. Believe me, you will probably end up thinking, "That's plenty!"

As I mentioned earlier, be sure to set yourself up for success. Block the time out on your schedule, have your workout clothes laid out, favorite workout playlists ready to pump you up, and have water close by.

Now, let's look at some new exercises to help you get healthier, fitter, and stronger!

Chapter 3 – Exercises

In this chapter, you'll see some new exercises that will be used in the workouts later in the book. Some will be bodyweight exercises, while others will use the equipment described earlier. As in my last book, there will be links to short videos that show exactly how to perform the exercises correctly. Hey, I like to make your learning process as easy as possible!

Jump Rope Variations

Many of my students have not jumped rope since they were kids! And that's fine. Just do the best you can. If Jump Rope work is still too challenging for you, then you can substitute Jumping Jacks, or even marching in place.

Single Unders

1. Stand with your feet a few inches apart. Hold the jump rope handles in each hand with the rope hanging to the floor behind you.
2. Swing the rope over your head and in front of you.
3. Jump up high enough so that the rope can pass underneath both feet at the same time. Keep your legs straight (more or less) as you jump.
4. Repeat, counting each time the rope passes beneath you as one rep.
5. Video – Jump Rope Variations

---------->

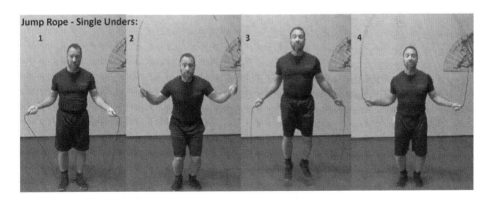

Jump Rope - Single Unders:

12

Single Unders – Running Step

1. Begin with regular Single Unders as depicted above.
2. Switch to a running step, hitting the floor with only one foot at a time in between each rope turn. Raise your knee high on each step. Count each time the rope passes beneath you as one rep, regardless of which foot was used.
3. Video – Jump Rope Variations

---------->

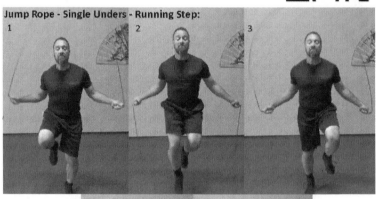

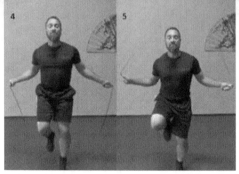

Jump Rope - Single Unders - Running Step:

Double Unders

1. Begin with regular Single Unders as depicted above.
2. Jump up high enough so that the rope can pass underneath both feet at the same time. Keep your legs straight (more or less) as you jump. Keep your hands close to your body and move the rope fast enough so that it goes under your feet twice for each jump. The motion should come from wrist action, not big arm swings, and the rope has to move *FAST*!!
3. Repeat, counting each time the rope passes twice beneath you as one rep. (I count each time my feet hit the ground.)

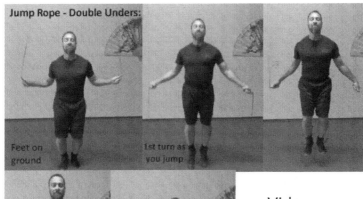

Jump Rope - Double Unders:

Feet on ground

1st turn as you jump

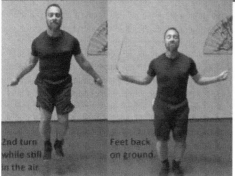

2nd turn while still in the air

Feet back on ground.

Video - Jump Rope Variations

14

Medicine Ball Squats

1. Stand with your feet shoulder-width apart. Hold the medicine ball at chest level, close to your body.

2. Bend your knees and lower your upper body until your thighs are at least parallel to the ground, ideally until the crease of your hips is below your knees. Keep your knees directly over your feet, head up, and back straight. Focus on putting all of your weight on your heels.

3. Then straighten your legs until you are standing straight and tall again.

4. Video: Medicine Ball Squats

------------------->

Medicine Ball Squats – cont'd

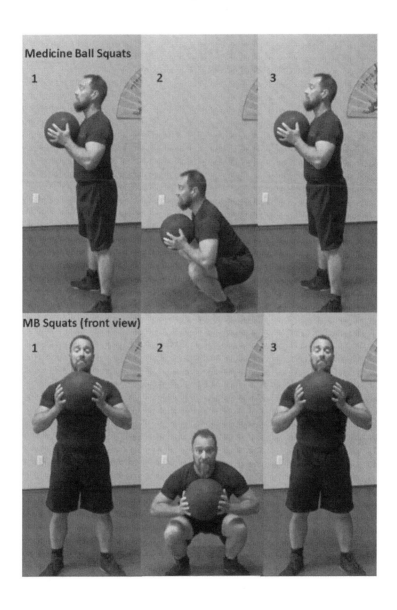

Woodchoppers

1. Stand with your feet shoulder-width apart. Hold the medicine ball at chest level, close to your body.
2. Bend your knees and lower your upper body until your thighs are at least parallel to the ground. Tap the medicine ball on the floor between your feet.
3. Curl your arms to bring the medicine ball back to your chest.
4. Straighten your legs explosively and launch yourself upwards: jump! As your legs straighten and you begin to jump, press the medicine ball straight up over your head as though you were trying to touch the ceiling with it.
5. As you come back to your feet, immediately drop back down into the next repetition.
6. Video: Woodchoppers

------------>

Woodchoppers – cont'd

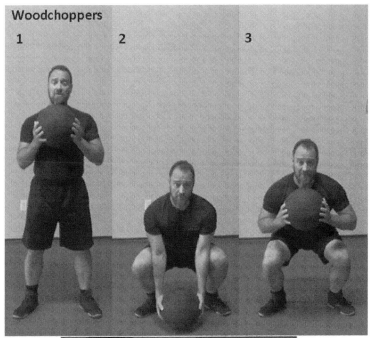

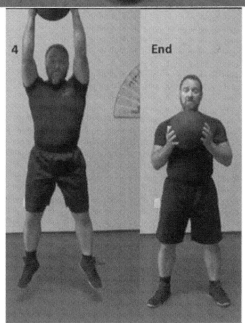

Divebomber Pushups

This is a challenging exercise that builds great upper body and core strength.

1. Stand with your feet a little wider than shoulder-width apart. Bend over until you can put your hands on the floor in front of you, just about shoulder-width apart. Walk your hands forward 6-10 inches.

2-3. Bend your elbows and lower your body towards the floor in an arcing motion. Pretend you are rolling a ball forward on the floor with your chest.

4. Complete the arc by straightening your arms, keep your hips down close to the floor, bring your head up and look at the ceiling.

5. Bend your elbows again and reverse the arc to go back to your starting position. When you have returned to the start, that is one rep.

6. Video – Divebombers and Hindu Pushups

------------->

Divebomber Pushups – Cont'd

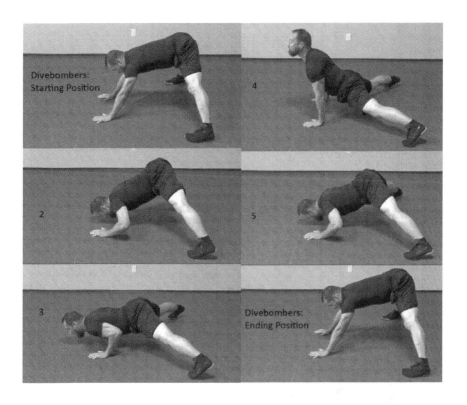

Divebombers: Starting Position

4

2

5

3

Divebombers: Ending Position

Alternate: **Hindu Pushups**

1. Begin in the same position as Divebomber Pushups.
2-4. Follow the same arc as in DB Pushups until your arms are straight and you are looking at the ceiling, hips close to the ground.
5. Rather than reversing the arc as in Divebomber Pushups, leave your arms straight and move your body back to the starting position.
6. Video – DiveBombers and Hindu Pushups

------------>

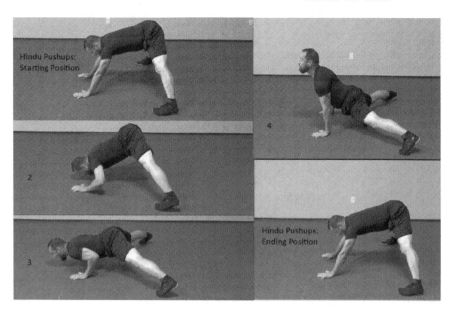

V-Ups

Another effective way to strengthen your abdominal muscles.

1. Lie on your back with your knees up and feet flat. Extend your arms over your head.
2. Bring your arms forward, tighten your stomach muscles, and raise your body towards your knees as if performing a Sit Up. Keeping your legs together, bring them up towards the ceiling. Strive to touch your feet or shins with your hands.
3. Lower yourself back to a lying position and bring your arms back to where they were.
4. Video – V-Ups --------->

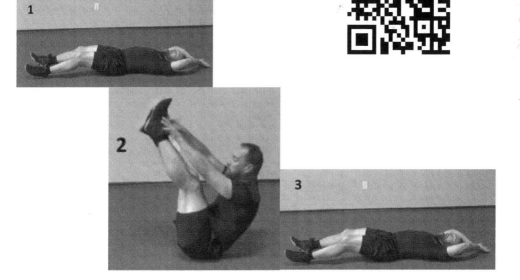

Chinnies

1. Lie on your back with your knees up and feet flat. Place your fingertips on your head behind your ears, and hold your elbows out to either side.

2. Tighten your stomach muscles, raise your chin, and raise your chest and shoulders up off the ground. Pick up your feet and extend your legs straight in front of you. Maintain a crunched position throughout the exercise.

3. Bring one knee towards your chest and crunch/twist the opposite elbow toward that knee.

4. Moving quickly, repeat the process on the opposite side.

5. Move rapidly back and forth between each side.

6. Video – Chinnies

----------->

Chinnies – cont'd

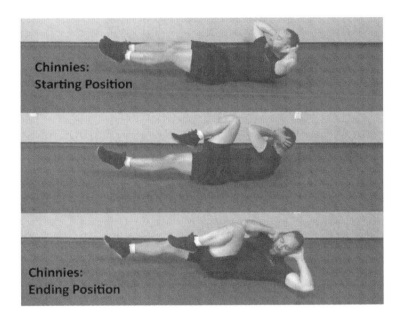

Chinnies:
Starting Position

Chinnies:
Ending Position

Medicine Ball Sit-Ups

Adding resistance to your sit-ups is a great way to increase your core strength.

1. Lie on your back with your knees up and feet flat. Hold a medicine ball on your chest, just under your chin.
2. Tighten your stomach muscles and raise your body towards your knees until you reach a sitting position. Hold the medicine ball in place.
3. Return to the starting position with your back on the floor.
4. Video – Med Ball Sit-Ups

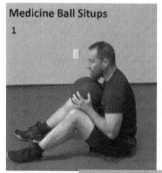

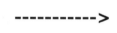 

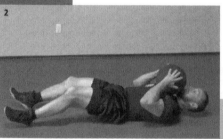

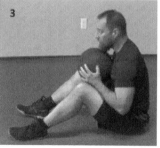

Pull-Ups

Pull-Ups are a really great for building strength in your arms, back, and core. They're also quite a challenge for most people, so get ready to have some fun! I'm assuming you're using a doorway-mounted pull-up bar as suggested earlier, but if you've gone the extra mile and bought a stand-alone bar or mounted one permanently somewhere, good for you! If you do use the doorway version, make sure it's properly installed and in good working order.

1. Reach up and grab the bar with your hands shoulder-width apart, palms facing away from you.
2. Bend your knees until your arms are straight and then pick your feet up off the floor. This is your starting position.
3. Pull yourself up until your chin is above the level of the bar.
4. Return to the starting position (feet off the floor, knees bent, arms straight)
5. Video – Pull-Ups, Jumping Pull-Ups, & Assisted Pull-Ups

------------>

Pull-Ups – Cont'd

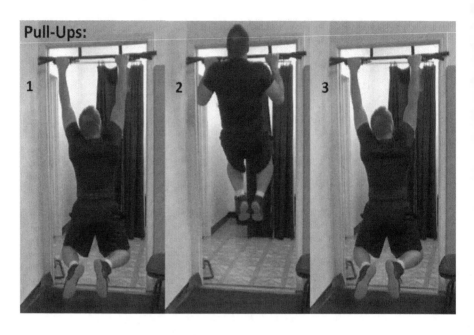

Pull-Ups:

Alternate - Jumping Pull-Ups

Pull-Ups are fabulous for building strength, but are really challenging if you're not used to them. Many folks are unable to do even one 'regular' pull-up. Jumping pull-ups are a great alternative, and an easier way to get started with this type of pulling exercise.

1. Reach up and grab the bar with your hands shoulder-width apart, palms facing away from you.
2. Keeping your feet flat on the floor, bend your knees until your arms are straight. This is your starting position.
3. Jump up and pull at the same time, trying to get your chin above the level of the bar.
4. Return to the starting position (feet on floor, knees bent, arms straight)

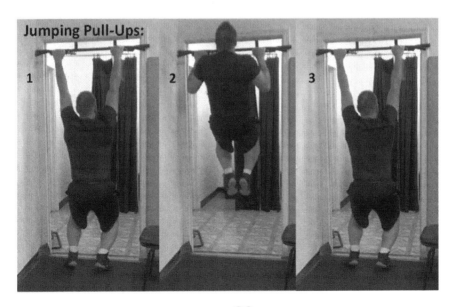

Jumping Pull-Ups:
1   2   3

Alternate - Assisted Pull-Ups

Although stretch bands are often used for assisted pull-ups, I'm going to show another option that you probably already have at home so that you don't have to buy another piece of equipment. As always, be careful!

1. Place a chair, stool, or sturdy box on the floor just behind where you will stand to begin your pullups.
2. Reach up and grab the bar with your hands shoulder-width apart, palms facing away from you.
3. Pick up your feet, one at a time, and place your shins or toes on the box/chair for support. Hang until your arms are straight. This is your starting position.
4. Pull yourself up until your chin is above the level of the bar. Rest as much weight as necessary on your legs or feet to allow you to complete the movement.
5. Return to the starting position (feet on floor, knees bent, arms straight)
6. Video – Pull-Ups, Jumping Pull-Ups, & Assisted Pull-Ups

----------->

Assisted Pull-Ups – Cont'd

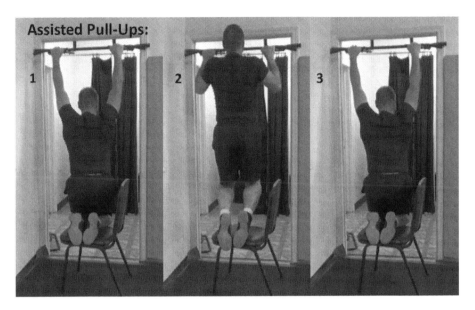

Assisted Pull-Ups:
1
2
3

Other Exercises

In the first book, we covered several fundamental exercises. Some of these will be sprinkled throughout the workouts later in this book; by now, you should know them like old friends! Just in case you need a refresher on any of these, follow the QR code to the JMMA YouTube channel.

Squats and variations
Lunges
Pushups
Sit Ups
Burpees
Jumping Jacks
Mountain Climbers
Running and Walking

Chapter 4 – Warm Ups and Workouts

Ok, you've got your workout clothes on, your water is close at hand, the music has got you revved up and ready to go, so what's left? The Warm Up!

It's very important to prepare your body for strenuous activity, and that's the truth for beginners and pro athletes alike. You've got to raise your body temperature and go through a series of motions to 'wake up' your body before you get into more strenuous training. I often choose to go for a short run (jog) and then go through the following movements before I get to work. I detailed this in the previous book, but it never hurts to see it again.

Oiling the Joints

At Jade Mountain Martial Arts, we have a short set of exercises that we often perform to get our bodies ready to train. We call it "Oiling the Joints." By moving our joints through their range of motion, synovial fluid is pumped into the joints. This lubricates and protects them for more rigorous motions. Our pattern starts at the top of the body and works downwards from there.

Neck: Gently turn your head left and right (as if you're saying 'no') 6 or 8 times. Next, tilt your head back and forth 6 or 8 times (as if you're saying 'yes'). Then tilt it side to side a few times (think of a dog when it hears a funny sound). Last, gently roll it to one side, then to the other.

Shoulders: Roll your shoulders forward a few times, then backwards. Next, twist one arm until your palm faces up, then turn and twist the other arm the same way. (We call it The Egyptian, after the old pictures in the pyramids) Repeat a few times on each side.

Waist: Letting your arms swing, twist your body to the left, then to the right. Repeat 5 or 10 times. Next, rotate your body as if you had a big Hula Hoop, first in one direction a few times, then the other.

Knees: Keep your knees together, and rotate them first one direction a few times, then repeat in the other direction.

Ankles: Trace the outline of one foot on the floor, keeping your knee still. Move first in one direction, then the other. Then repeat with the other foot.

Video – Oiling the Joints --->

Now that you've Oiled the Joints, it's a good idea to do a few repetitions of the exercises that you'll be using in whatever workout you choose. Just a few repetitions of each exercise will suffice, then you can get started.

Types of Workouts

Let's review the different types of workouts that you'll see in the next section.

AMRAP

This stands for **A**s **M**any **R**ounds (or **R**epetitions) **A**s **P**ossible. I love running workouts like these because they allow people of very different fitness levels to train simultaneously and everyone gets a great workout! Some super-fit folks might do 15 rounds of work while newer folks might only get 5, but in an AMRAP, everyone gets an opportunity to get a workout that's right for them. By now, you should know how your body responds and might be ready to push a little harder!

X Rounds For Time (RFT)

This stands for a set amount of work that you will try to accomplish. Some folks will complete a workout of 5 rounds of 10 reps each of several exercises in just a few minutes, while others take much longer. Whatever your time, just strive to be correct in your technique and go as fast as you safely can. Mark your time and then try to beat it next time!

Circuit

A Circuit is a workout in which you will be doing several different exercises. Starting with one exercise, you will do as many repetitions of that exercises as you can for a set amount of time. Then you switch to the next exercise, and do the same thing. As each time interval passes, you move to the next exercise until you have performed all of the exercises in the workout. That is one round. You can do as many rounds as you decide, or however many the workout calls for.

A Word of Caution!!

If you've already been working out with the first book, then you've likely achieved a better understanding of your body. By now, you know how hard is 'too hard', and have a good idea what your body can do and how fast. You're not a newbie anymore. Nevertheless, **don't overdo it!** If you feel sharp pains in any of your joints or muscles, or if you start seeing pretty little sparkles in front of your eyes, **STOP!** Although I want you to begin pushing harder and being determined, there's no need to hurt yourself, pass out, or throw up from a workout. Those things are not badges of honor...they are often signs of knuckleheadedness. Be smart, work hard, challenge yourself, but don't damage yourself for the sake of a few seconds on the clock or a few more reps on the board.

Now that we've discussed safety and the different types of workouts, let's get to work!

WORKOUTS

1. Fifty Shades of Sweaty (AMRAP) – 15 minutes

        10 Woodchoppers
        10 V-Ups
        10 Divebomber Pushups
        10 Pullups
        10 Burpees

Do 10 of each exercise, then move to the next exercise until you've done all five, then start another round. Keep track of how many total rounds you complete, plus how many reps into the final round. Modify the exercises (use alternates) as necessary.

2. Minute Drills (Circuit) – 5 rounds

Jump Rope (SU's or DU's)	1 minute
Pushups	1 minute
Med Ball Squats	1 minute
Chinnies	1 minute

Keep a close eye on your timer! Transition as quickly as you can in between exercises and hang in there!

3. Pullups, V-Ups, and MB Squats (RFT) – 5 rounds

10 Pullups
15 V-Ups
20 Medicine Ball Squats

Keep track of how long it takes you to get through all five rounds. Rest as little as possible, but as much as you need to. Just keep at it, rep by rep, until you get through the whole thing, even if you have to take extra time to do it. That said, I always want you to listen to your body, and if you experience sharp pains anywhere, then stop!

4. 150 Burpees for Time! – 1 round

150 Burpees

At my school, Jade Mountain Martial Arts, we do the 100 Burpee workout every so often as a benchmark. Many folks have their times marked down so they can track their progress. When they start getting down to the 6-7 minute range, I throw this workout at them. It's both a physical challenge and a mental one. When you get all the way through this, I bet you'll feel like everything else in your life seems a little easier. Give it a shot, you might surprise yourself!

5. 1000 Double Unders For Time – 1 round

1000 Double Unders

You read that correctly. I do this workout myself every once in a while because it's definitely a challenge! It will also help you improve your jump rope technique just because of the amount of practice you get. Keep track of how long it takes you to get through it, and next time, try and beat your time. You can also do this with Single Unders if DU's are not yet in your skill set. If you do choose SU's, then vary your jumping pattern. The variety makes it more fun!

Whether you're doing Doubles or Singles, it can be hard to keep track of so many reps, especially when you start to get tired. I always lay out ten coins on the floor, then slide one away from the others each time I reach 100 reps. It's a great visual reference to keep you on track.

6. On The Floor, But More! (AMRAP) – 15 Minutes

10 Mountain Climbers (left, right, equals 1)
10 Divebomber Pushups
10 Mountain Climbers (left, right, equals 1)
10 V-Ups

You might want to lay a towel on the floor for this one. Start the timer and get to work! Note how many times you can get through the series.

7. PPS (AMRAP) – 15-20 Minutes

5 Jumping Pull-ups	5 Pull-ups
10 Pushups	10 Divebomber pushups
15 Squats	15 Medicine Ball Squats

I've listed two different versions of this one: one that's easier and then a more challenging set. Choose your time, 15 or 20 minutes, then choose which version you want to do. Keep track of how many complete sets (and the reps from your last set too, if it was incomplete) so you can try to beat it next time.

8. Deck of Doom (or Victory) II! (RFT) – 1 round

      This is another version of a workout described in the first book, but this time, it's a bit more challenging! For this workout, you'll need an ordinary deck of playing cards. Shuffle them well! Now, let's assign some more difficult exercises to each suit.

Hearts   -   Burpees
Diamonds -   Divebomber Pushups
Spades   -   Woodchoppers
Clubs   -   V-Ups

      The number on the card tells you how many reps of each exercise to do. Face cards count as 10 repetitions. The Aces can be either 1 rep or (if you're feeling sturdy) 11 reps. Jokers can either be discarded or Wild! Pick another exercise such as 50 Jumping Jacks or if you have the available space, a short sprint! Turn the first card over, do the designated number of reps for that exercise, then go to the next card.

      You can use a stopwatch to time yourself as you work your way through the deck, go as fast as you can! You can leave the cards unshuffled after your workout and try it again sometime later and see if you can beat your time! Or you can shuffle the deck for a new workout. For even more variety, change the exercises. There are many possibilities with this particular workout so don't be afraid to change it up and then push yourself to see what you can do!

9. 30-25-20 (Circuit) – 3 rounds

Round 1	Round 2	Round 3
30 Double Unders	25 D-U's	20 D-U's
30 Pushups	25 Pushups	20 Pushups
30 Pull-ups	25 Pull-ups	20 Pull-ups

This workout is 3 rounds, and the number of reps for each exercise diminishes each round. Try and push hard through all three rounds, knowing that the rounds get shorter each time. If you get through this one and feel like you want more of a challenge, change the rep sets to 50-30-20 next time and have even more sweaty fun!

Chapter 5 – Workouts with Running

Running and walking are great ways to improve your overall health, and since we discussed some simple ways to get started in the last book, I'm going to assume that you've done some walking, jogging, and maybe running since then. By now, you know what a great workout it can be, whatever your fitness level. If a brisk walk is all you can handle, then walk it out! If you can run or jog, but only for short distances, then that's great! Just keep it up!

Since we're taking things a step farther in this book, I'll give you some new workouts that add running into the mix. You will want to have a safe route planned ahead of time to run for various distances. I use http://www.mapmyrun.com as an easy way to plan my routes. Dress appropriately for the weather, and keep your eyes open so you don't trip or run into traffic!

#1 – 12-24-36-400m (RFT) – 4 rounds

12 Burpees
24 Pushups
36 Squats
400m Run

This one is a ton of sweaty fun! Each round starts with calisthenics, then ends with a 400m run (that's one lap around a standard high school or college track, but I have a route in my subdivision that covers the same distance and starts/ends in my driveway).

#2 – 21-15-9-400m (RFT) – 3 rounds

Although it has fewer rounds than the first workout, this one can be a real challenge! This time, you'll start with the run...and run as fast as you can!

400m Run

Woodchoppers

Pull-ups

The first round, you'll run 400m, then do 21 Woodchoppers and 21 Pull-ups (strict, assisted, or jumping, whatever you are capable of performing). On the second round, you'll run first, then only do 15 Woodchoppers and 15 Pull-ups. On the last round, you'll run and then finish up with only 9 Woodchoppers and 9 Pull-ups. Done!

Try to push hard throughout the workout, knowing that each successive round will have fewer repetitions for you to deal with!

#3 – Running for Distance

You might have already started some running after reading the first book. When doing these same workouts now, you might find that your time has improved or that you don't have to walk as often (or at all!) during your longer runs. As before, keep track of your times so that you can see your progress. And don't worry if you don't improve your times every single workout. Not every time will be a personal best, and that's totally ok. You're getting healthier and stronger from doing consistent workouts, and that's what's important!

½ mile (800m) – 2 laps around an official high school/college track.
1 mile (1600m) – 4 laps
2 miles (3200m) – 8 laps
5K – (5000m) – 3.1 miles, or a little more than 12 laps
10K – (10,000m) – 6.2 miles

Whether you run the whole way, walk it instead, or a combination of both, running is extremely beneficial.

#4 – Sprints!

Sprints are great metabolism boosters, and will really improve your overall conditioning. They're a real challenge, though, so be prepared to work! Make sure you warm up thoroughly before attempting any kind of sprints, as they require your body to be working at its maximum effort, whatever that may be.

10 to 20 – 40 yard sprints with a 30 second rest. Maximum effort!

If you have access to a track, another good sprint workout is as follows:

Sprint the straightaways
Jog (or Walk) the curves. Do this for as many laps as you choose.

#5 – Fartlek Running

One more that I enjoy is a lot more variable, but that makes it fun! It's got a funny name, but hey, it is what it is.

This workout is best done over a longer time period, say 40 minutes to an hour of running. The trick is to vary your running speed throughout the course. Sprint a bit, then jog, then run faster, then jog, then sprint again, then slow down again. The key is to just keep moving. Change up your pace whenever you feel like it, and throw some good, sturdy sprints in there. And remember, you do not have to match anyone else's speed...it's all you, my friend. Just do what you can do, see how your body responds, and then figure out when you're ready to push harder. It's all good.

Chapter 6 – Summing It Up

By now, you should have built a habit of working out. You might even be looking forward to each training session!

Once you have laid that foundation of fitness and have a better understanding of how your body responds, you can really start to push harder and make even more progress.

The goal at this point should be to be as consistent as possible in terms of how many days a week you train. Striving for three to five workouts a week is a good plan, and you can always take a rest day whenever you feel the need; just get back on track as quickly as possible! Consistency over time truly makes the difference. The way I see it, the time is going to pass anyway, and you may as well spend a tiny piece of each day doing something that will help you live a healthier and happier life.

A year from now, you can look back over the past year and either say, *"Dang, I wish I had done something to get in shape...I hate feeling weak and sick all the time,"* or you can look back and say, *"Wow, when I started exercising, I couldn't even jog a quarter of a mile, and now I'm running in a 5K for fun! I feel great!"* I hear comments like these often in my line of work, so I know it's not science fiction. It just takes a plan, some time, and some energy, and then great things happen.

Try the workouts in this book and see how they work for you. If you have questions or need some encouragement, I'm always just an email away!

The End

Afterword

In this book, we took it up a notch. You've learned a few new ways to exercise with a few versatile pieces of equipment. I enjoy adding different elements to my workouts because they challenge me and keep things interesting. Also, it's important to utilize different movements so that you will be stronger in a wider range of positions and situations...if all you ever do is the bench press, you'll likely have fabulous pecs, but might be underconditioned in every other part of your body! So mix it up, have some fun, and enjoy getting healthier and stronger!

To be notified of other books in the Jade Mountain Workout Series when they are published, sign up for our mailing list at www.jmma.org!

About The Author

Sifu Whit McClendon was born on October 31, 1969 in Freeport, Tx. He grew up in Angleton Texas and was active in martial arts, track and field, and playing the clarinet in band. After working in the petrochemical field as a CAD drafter for many years, Whit finally realized his life's dream of becoming a full-time martial arts instructor. He now lives with his family in Katy, Texas, plays lacrosse as often as possible, and runs Jade Mountain Martial Arts. He is also an author of fantasy novels, which can be found at http://www.jidaan.com.

Whit has intensively studied Kung Fu, Krav Maga, Taiji, Kickboxing, and Brazilian Jiu Jitsu since 1982. He has been a CrossFit Lvl 1 certified Coach, a level 2 Kettlebell instructor, and is well-versed in the techniques and applications of cardio & resistance training. He is a CrossFit Games competitor, a 2 time National AAU Shuai Jiao silver medalist, a Tough Mudder enthusiast, lacrosse player, and a 4 time Houston Half-Marathon Finisher.

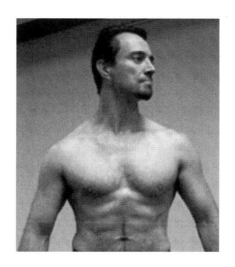

whitmcc@jmma.org

www.jmma.org

www.whitmcclendon.com

Made in the USA
Coppell, TX
11 January 2020